# Low Lectin Diet

Adopting A Low Lectin Diet to Nourish Your Body and Health for Maximum Wellness

**Anne Finley**

Copyright © 2023

## All Rights Are Reserved

The content in this book may not be reproduced, duplicated, or transferred without the express written permission of the author or publisher. Under no circumstances will the publisher or author be held liable or legally responsible for any losses, expenditures, or damages incurred directly or indirectly as a consequence of the information included in this book.

## Legal Remarks

**Copyright protection applies to this publication. It is only intended for** personal use. No piece of this work may be modified, distributed, sold, quoted, or paraphrased without the author's or publisher's consent.

## Disclaimer Statement

Please keep in mind that the contents of this booklet are meant for educational and recreational purposes. Every effort has been made to offer accurate, up-to-date, reliable, and thorough information. There are, however, no stated or implied assurances of any kind. Readers understand that the author is providing competent counsel. The content in this book originates from several sources. Please seek the opinion of a competent professional before using any of the tactics outlined in this book. By reading this book, the reader agrees that the author will not be held accountable for any direct or indirect damages resulting from the use of the information contained therein, including, but not limited to, errors, omissions, or inaccuracies.

# TABLE OF CONTENTS

# INTRODUCTION

Welcome to the Low Lectin Diet, a revolutionary approach to nourishing your body and revitalizing your health. In today's fast-paced world, processed and convenience foods dominate our plates, exposing us to substances that disrupt our body's delicate balance. Lectins, a group of proteins found in many plant-based foods, have been associated with various health concerns. This comprehensive guide aims to dispel myths about lectins and provide you with the knowledge and strategies to navigate a low lectin diet successfully.

The book combines scientifically-backed research and practical insights from over 30 years of experience in promoting health and well-being. It takes you on a journey of self-discovery, exploring the science of lectin sensitivity and its impact on digestion, inflammation, and overall health. Armed with this knowledge, you can make informed decisions about your dietary habits and unlock the door to a healthier, more vibrant life.

The Low Lectin Diet promotes a balanced and thoughtful approach to adopting a reduced-lectin diet. You will learn to identify high-lectin foods and reduce their presence in your meals without sacrificing taste or satisfaction. By embracing a low lectin diet, you can nourish your body with nutrient-dense, low-inflammatory foods that support optimal health.

Transitioning to a low lectin diet may seem challenging, but the book provides practical tips and guidance to help you get started. From pantry makeovers to grocery shopping advice, you will have the tools to transform your kitchen into a health sanctuary. With comprehensive meal plans, delicious recipes, and cooking techniques that reduce lectin content, you will be inspired to create wholesome and flavourful meals.

The book recognizes the importance of customization and offers guidance for adapting the low lectin diet to different dietary preferences and lifestyles. Whether you are a vegetarian, vegan, or have specific dietary requirements, you can tailor the diet to suit your needs.

The Low Lectin Diet goes beyond food and explores the role of key nutrients, supplements, stress management, sleep, exercise, and alternative health practices. It provides practical solutions for dining out and navigating social situations while following the diet.

Embracing a low lectin diet is a transformative journey, and the book emphasizes the importance of patience, self-compassion, and an open mind. The benefits are numerous, including improved digestion, weight management, reduced inflammation, enhanced immune function, and increased vitality.

This book is your trusted companion on the path to embracing a low lectin diet. It empowers you to take control of your health, make informed choices, and experience a profound shift in your well-being. Let us embark on this life-changing journey together, nurturing our bodies and minds with the wisdom and insights within these pages.

# CHAPTER ONE

## Exploring Lectin Sensitivity

## Identifying Lectin Sensitivity Symptoms

Identifying Lectin Sensitivity Symptoms

Lectin sensitivity is defined by an individual's negative responses to lectin-rich meals. While lectins are found in many plant-based meals, not everyone develops lectin sensitivity symptoms. Those that do, however, will find that understanding the signals is critical in regulating their diet and general health. Here are some of the most prevalent signs of lectin sensitivity:

**1. Digestive pain:** Digestive pain is a common sign of lectin sensitivity. Bloating, gas, stomach discomfort, cramps, diarrhea, or constipation are all symptoms of this. These symptoms arise as a result of lectin contact with the digestive tract lining, which may result in inflammation and disruption of normal gut function.

**2. Joint Pain and Inflammation:** In certain people, lectins have been related to joint pain and inflammation. Lectins may cause an immunological response, resulting in joint inflammation, stiffness, swelling, and pain.

**3. Skin Problems:** Lectin sensitivity has been linked to a variety of skin disorders such as rashes, eczema, acne, and psoriasis. Lectins may lead to increased skin inflammation and aggravate pre-existing skin problems in some situations.

**4. Fatigue and Low Energy:** Lectin sensitivity can cause fatigue and low energy levels. The immune system's reaction to lectins may result in a systemic inflammatory response, leaving people fatigued and depleted of energy.

**5. Brain Fog and Cognitive Issues:** Lectins have the capacity to breach the blood-brain barrier and disrupt brain function. Some people who are sensitive to lectins may have brain fog, trouble concentrating, memory issues, or cognitive impairment.

**6. Autoimmune Symptoms:** Lectins have been linked to the initiation or exacerbation of autoimmune disorders. Consuming lectin-rich foods may cause an increase in symptoms such as joint pain, inflammation, exhaustion, and digestive difficulties in people who already have autoimmune illnesses.

**7.Allergic Reactions**: Lectins can cause allergic reactions such as hives, swelling, itching, or trouble breathing in rare situations. Individuals with a documented allergy to certain lectin-containing foods are more likely to have these symptoms.

## How Lectins Affect Digestion and Gut Health

Lectins, a kind of protein present in a variety of plant-based meals, have been shown to improve digestion and gut health. Understanding how lectins impact these processes is critical for those who want to improve their digestive function and general health. The following is an explanation of how lectins affect digestion and gut health:

**1. Intestinal Barrier Integrity:** The intestinal lining works as a protective barrier, selectively enabling nutrients to be absorbed while keeping dangerous things out. Lectins can attach to certain carbohydrates on the surface of intestinal cells, possibly affecting the barrier's integrity. When lectins attach to these cells, they can induce cellular damage and inflammation and disrupt the tight junctions that connect the intestinal cells.

This can result in increased intestinal permeability, often known as "leaky gut syndrome." A leaky gut allows undigested food particles, poisons, and germs to enter the circulation, activating immunological responses and potentially leading to digestive disorders and systemic inflammation.

**2. Inhibition of Enzymes:** Lectins can inhibit the functioning of some digestive enzymes. These enzymes are in charge of converting carbs, proteins, and lipids into smaller, more absorbable components. Incomplete digestion and poor nutrient absorption can occur when lectins block these enzymes. This can lead to vitamin shortages and bodily imbalances.

**3: Disruption of the Gut Microbiota:** The gut microbiota, a complex colony of bacteria living in the intestines, plays an important role in digestion and general health. Lectins have a direct influence on the makeup and diversity of the gut microbiota. Some lectins have been demonstrated to attach to the surface of particular bacteria, affecting their growth patterns and potentially disturbing the microbiota's delicate equilibrium. This imbalance can result in dysbiosis, which is characterized by an imbalance of dangerous and good bacteria and is linked to a variety of digestive diseases and immune system malfunctions.

**4. Inflammation:** Lectins have been linked to increased inflammation in the digestive tract. When lectins attach to intestinal cells, an immunological response is triggered, resulting in the production of pro-inflammatory chemicals. Chronic gut inflammation can lead to the development of digestive illnesses such as inflammatory bowel disease (IBD), irritable bowel syndrome (IBS), and other gastrointestinal disorders.

**5. Lectin Sensitivity:** Some people are more sensitive to lectins than others. Lectin sensitivity refers to the unfavorable effects that people may have when they consume lectin-rich foods. These responses can range from moderate digestive discomfort, such as bloating and gas, to more severe symptoms, such as stomach pain, diarrhea, and inflammation. Lectin sensitivity is assumed to be caused by a combination of genetic predisposition, individual immune system responses, and the amount and kind of lectins eaten.

**Managing Lectin's Impact on Digestion and Gut Health:**

- **Cooking and processing:** Certain foods can be reduced in lectin concentration and digestibility by cooking, soaking, fermenting, or sprouting.
- **Variety and moderation:** Eating a variety of plant-based meals will help reduce lectin exposure while

still reaping nutritional advantages. Consuming lectin-rich foods in moderation may also be advantageous for people who are sensitive to them.

- **Gut-supportive practices:** Prioritizing a fiber-rich, prebiotic-rich, and probiotic-rich diet can help support a healthy gut flora and promote optimum digestion.

- **Individualization:** Recognizing one's unique lectin sensitivity and collaborating with healthcare specialists such as registered dietitians or functional medicine practitioners can assist in tailoring an optimal dietary plan that addresses individual needs and improves gut health.

## Lectins and Inflammation

Lectins, a protein group present in a variety of plant-based foods, have been linked to inflammation in the body. Inflammation is the immune system's natural response to protect itself from damage, infection, or foreign chemicals. When inflammation becomes chronic or severe, it can lead to the development of a variety of health problems. In this in-depth discussion, we will look at the link between lectins and inflammation, specifically how lectins may cause or increase inflammatory reactions in the body.

**1. Lectin Properties and Interactions:** Lectins are carbohydrate-binding proteins that can detect and attach to particular sugar molecules on the cell surface. This binding can happen in a variety of tissues and organs throughout the body, such as the digestive system, blood vessels, and immune cells. Lectins can bind to cell membranes and activate signaling pathways that regulate immune responses and inflammation.

**2. Lectins and immunological Activation:** Lectins can activate immunological responses when they attach to the surface of cells. Immune cells, such as macrophages and lymphocytes, are activated, releasing pro-inflammatory chemicals such as cytokines and chemokines. These chemicals cause inflammation and attract extra immune cells to the lectin interaction site. NF-B and other inflammatory signaling pathways are frequently engaged in lectin-mediated immune activation and subsequent inflammation.

**3. Gut Inflammation and Lectins:** Due to the high concentration of lectins in many plant-based meals, the gut is particularly vulnerable to lectin-mediated inflammation. Lectins have the potential to adhere to the intestinal lining, compromising the integrity of the intestinal barrier and resulting in increased intestinal permeability, often known as leaky gut. This lets hazardous items into the circulation, such as germs, poisons, and undigested food particles. When the immune system detects these intruders, it initiates an inflammatory reaction.

Inflammatory bowel disease (IBD) and irritable bowel syndrome (IBS) have been related to chronic gut inflammation caused by lectin exposure.

**4. Autoimmune Diseases and Lectins:**

Autoimmune illnesses develop when the immune system assaults its own tissues, resulting in persistent inflammation. Lectins have been linked to the development or worsening of autoimmune disorders. When lectin binds to cells in numerous organs, an immunological response is triggered, resulting in inflammation and tissue damage. For example, lectins may contribute to inflammation and aggravate symptoms in autoimmune disorders such as rheumatoid arthritis, lupus, and celiac disease.

**5. Lectin Sensitivity and Inflammation:** Some people are more sensitive to lectins than others, resulting in unpleasant responses and increased inflammation when exposed to lectins.

Lectin sensitivity can cause gastrointestinal problems, joint discomfort, skin problems, exhaustion, and other inflammatory symptoms. Reduced lectin consumption or adopting a low-lectin diet may help relieve symptoms and reduce inflammation in some circumstances.

**6. Cooking, Processing, and Lectin Activity:** Cooking, soaking, fermenting, or sprouting specific foods can help lower lectin activity and make them more palatable for lectin-sensitive persons. Heat and specific food processing methods can destroy or neutralize lectins, lowering their ability to cause inflammation. It is crucial to remember, however, that not all lectins are completely removed by boiling or processing, and sensitivity might still differ across individuals.

**7. Individual Variability and Lectin Tolerance:** It is critical to understand that lectin sensitivity and tolerance differ between individuals. While some people may have severe inflammation and unfavorable responses to lectins, others may tolerate them with no obvious effects.

A person's reaction to lectin exposure can be influenced by factors such as heredity, gastrointestinal health, immune system function, and overall nutrition.

**Managing Lectin-Induced Inflammation:**

- **Adopting a Low-Lectin Diet:** Adopting a low-lectin diet may be useful for persons with lectin sensitivity or conditions affected by lectins. This entails limiting or eliminating foods rich in lectins, such as legumes, nightshade vegetables, cereals, and some seeds.

- **Highlighting anti-inflammatory foods:** A nutritious diet rich in anti-inflammatory foods, such as fruits and vegetables, healthy fats, and lean meats, can help offset the inflammatory effects of lectins and improve general health.

- **Promoting gut health:** Consuming prebiotic and probiotic-rich foods can help promote a balanced immune response and reduce inflammation by maintaining a healthy gut microbiome.

# CHAPTER TWO

# THE BENEFITS OF A LOW LECTIN DIET

## Weight Management and Metabolism

Understanding the Relationship Between Metabolism and Weight Management

Metabolism refers to the complicated series of chemical processes that occur within living organisms in order to sustain life. It is the process through which food and nutrients are converted into energy and the building blocks required for growth, repair, and critical body processes. When it comes to weight loss, metabolism is important since it determines how effectively the body burns calories and stores or utilizes energy. Understanding the relationship between metabolism and weight management is critical for achieving and maintaining a healthy body weight and overall well-being.

**1. Basal Metabolic Rate (BMR):** The quantity of energy or calories required by the body to maintain vital activities at rest is known as the basal metabolic rate (BMR). These duties include breathing, circulating blood, controlling body temperature, and assisting important organs in their activities. BMR provides for the vast majority of total calories expended by the body each day, accounting for

60–75% of total energy expenditure. Age, gender, physical size, and heredity all have an impact on an individual's BMR.

**2. Thermic Effect of Food (TEF):** The energy used during the process of digesting, absorbing, and metabolizing nutrients from the food we eat is referred to as the thermic Effect of food. The body expends energy to convert macronutrients such as carbs, proteins, and fats into useable forms, which contributes to overall calorie expenditure. Protein has the greatest thermogenic impact, followed by carbs and fats. Consuming a well-balanced meal rich in protein might somewhat raise metabolism due to the extra energy required for digestion.

**3. Physical Activity:** Exercise and physical activity have a major influence on metabolism and weight control. Physical activities such as walking, jogging, strength training, and other types of exercise add to total daily energy expenditure. Regular exercise can boost metabolism by developing muscle mass, which requires more energy to maintain than fat tissue. Furthermore, high-intensity exercise can cause an "afterburn" effect, in which the body continues to burn calories at a high rate after activity.

Non-Exercise Activity

**4 non-Exercise activities Thermogenesis (NEAT):** The energy used during non-exercise activities such as fidgeting, standing, walking, and other everyday motions that are not scheduled workouts is referred to as thermogenesis (NEAT). NEAT varies greatly across people and influences total calorie expenditure.

Increasing NEAT by adding more activity to everyday activities can help with weight loss.

**5.Hormones and Metabolism:** Hormones have an important role in metabolism and weight management. Insulin, thyroid hormones, leptin, and ghrelin are hormones that impact hunger, fat storage, and energy expenditure. Insulin, for example, regulates blood sugar levels and encourages fat accumulation, whereas thyroid hormones control metabolism and energy generation. These hormone imbalances can have an influence on weight control and general health.

**6. Caloric Intake and Weight Control:** Caloric intake has an impact on weight control. When a person consumes more calories than their body expends, the surplus energy is stored as fat, resulting in weight gain. If caloric intake is less than energy expenditure, the body will burn stored fat for energy, resulting in weight loss. As a result, generating a calorie deficit through a mix of mindful eating and increased physical activity is frequently the primary weight reduction strategy.

**7. Individual Differences:** It is critical to understand that metabolism and weight control differ across individuals owing to genetic variables, age, body composition, hormone variations, and lifestyle behaviors. Some people's metabolisms are naturally quicker or slower than others. This can affect how their bodies adapt to calorie intake and expenditure.

**Tips for Healthy Weight Management:**

**1. Eat a well-balanced diet:**

Consume a wide range of nutrient-dense foods, such as whole grains, lean proteins, fruits and vegetables, and healthy fats.

**2. Regular physical activity:** Aim for a mix of aerobic, strength, and flexibility activities to improve overall fitness and metabolism.

**3. Practicing portion control:** Watch your portion sizes and pay attention to your body's hunger and fullness cues.

**4. Making sleep a priority:** Adequate sleep is necessary for hormone control and overall well-being.

**5.Stress management:** Because chronic stress can affect metabolism and weight control, adopt stress-relieving activities like meditation, yoga, or indulging in hobbies.

## Improve Digestion and Gut Health

Proper digestion and gut health are critical for overall health and vigor. As a nutritionist, I understand the critical role that diet plays in fostering healthy digestion and gut health. In this conversation, I'll go over major tactics and nutritional suggestions for improving digestion and cultivating a healthy gut microbiome.

**1. A Fiber-Rich and Balanced Diet:** Consuming a balanced diet that includes a range of whole foods is essential for healthier digestion. Incorporate a variety of fruits, vegetables, whole grains, lean meats, and healthy fats into your diet. Additionally, dietary fiber should be prioritized since it promotes regular bowel movements, avoids constipation, and maintains a healthy gut microbiome. Include high-fiber foods like legumes, whole grains, nuts, seeds, and lots of fruits and veggies in your everyday meals.

**2. Adequate Hydration:** Staying hydrated is critical for digestion. Water softens feces and facilitates their transit through the digestive tract. It also promotes the development of digestive enzymes, allowing for more effective nutritional digestion and absorption. Drink plenty of water throughout the day and think about including hydrating foods like cucumbers, melons, and leafy greens in your diet.

**3.Mindful Eating:** Mindful eating practices can dramatically improve digestion. Slow down and appreciate each bite, properly chewing food before swallowing. This promotes the mechanical digestion of food and the release of digestive enzymes in the mouth. Furthermore, mindful eating improves digestion by helping you tune in to your body's hunger and fullness cues, minimizing overeating and discomfort.

**4. Probiotics and Fermented Foods:** Consuming probiotics and fermented foods can help maintain a healthy gut microbiome. Probiotics are helpful microorganisms that aid digestion and help maintain a healthy gut ecology. Probiotics can be found in fermented foods such as yogurt, kefir, sauerkraut, kimchi, and tempeh. Consider including these foods in your diet on a regular basis, or look into high-quality probiotic supplements.

**5. Limit Processed and Added Sugars:** Processed meals, as well as those heavy in added sugars, can disturb gut health and cause digestive disorders. These meals are frequently poor in fiber and deficient in vital nutrients, which can impair digestion and increase inflammation in the stomach. When feasible, choose whole, unprocessed meals and minimize your intake of sugary snacks, sugary beverages, and highly processed foods.

**6. Manage Stress:** Stress may have a negative influence on digestion and gut health. When we are stressed, our bodies go into "fight-or-flight" mode, diverting resources away from digestion. This might cause symptoms including indigestion, bloating, and irregular bowel movements. Stress management approaches such as meditation, deep breathing exercises, regular physical activity, and making time for relaxation can all help with digestion.

**7. Determine Food Sensitivities:** Some people have food sensitivities or intolerances that might interfere with digestion. Lactose, gluten, and particular FODMAPs (fermentable oligosaccharides, disaccharides, monosaccharides, and polyols) are common causes. If you feel you have food sensitivities, consult with a certified dietitian who can assist you in identifying problem foods and developing a specific elimination diet or modification plan.

## Reduced Inflammation and Joint Pain

Understanding the Relationship Between Reduced Inflammation and Joint Pain

Inflammation is a normal immune system reaction to defend the body from damage, infection, or external invaders. When inflammation becomes chronic or severe, it can cause a variety of health problems, including joint pain and discomfort. Understanding the relationship between inflammation and joint pain is critical for treating and lowering discomfort in those who suffer from it. In this section, we will look at significant variables and solutions for lowering inflammation and joint discomfort.

**1. Inflammatory Conditions and Joint Pain:** Rheumatoid arthritis, osteoarthritis, gout, and autoimmune illnesses can all cause joint pain and inflammation. The immune system incorrectly assaults healthy tissues in these circumstances, resulting in persistent inflammation and joint degeneration. It is critical to collaborate with healthcare specialists, such as rheumatologists.

**2. Diet and Inflammation:** Diet is important in treating inflammation and joint discomfort. Certain meals can increase or decrease inflammation in the body. An anti-inflammatory diet can help relieve joint discomfort. Consume antioxidant-rich foods such as fruits, vegetables, whole grains, and healthy fats such as omega-3 fatty acids found in fatty fish, flaxseeds, and chia seeds. These nutrients aid in the fight against oxidative stress and inflammation.

**3. Omega-3 Fatty Acids:** Omega-3 fatty acids have anti-inflammatory qualities and may aid in the relief of joint discomfort. Include omega-3-rich foods in your diet, such as fatty fish (salmon, mackerel, and sardines), walnuts, flaxseeds, and chia seeds. Alternatively, in collaboration with a healthcare expert, omega-3 supplements may be advised.

**4. Maintaining a Healthy Weight:** Maintaining a healthy weight is essential for controlling joint pain and minimizing inflammation. Excess weight puts additional strain on joints, resulting in increased inflammation and pain.

Losing weight with a healthy diet and regular exercise can help relieve joint discomfort, especially in weight-bearing joints like the knees and hips.

**5. Physical Activity and Exercise:** Regular physical activity and exercise are crucial for joint health. Low-impact workouts such as walking, swimming, cycling, and light weight training can help strengthen the muscles around the joints, increase flexibility, and minimize joint discomfort. Consult a healthcare practitioner or a trained fitness expert to build an activity plan that is specific to your requirements and abilities.

Heat and ice treatments can both give brief relief from joint pain and inflammation. A warm compress or a warm bath can help relax muscles and enhance blood circulation to afflicted joints, relieving discomfort and stiffness. Ice packs or cold compresses, for example, can help numb the region and decrease inflammation. Alternate heat and cold treatments as directed by your healthcare provider.

**7. Stress Management and Rest:** Chronic stress can increase joint pain and inflammation. Stress management practices such as relaxation exercises, meditation, yoga, and engaging in activities that you love can help reduce stress and increase general well-being. Furthermore, getting enough rest and quality sleep helps the body's natural healing processes and relieves joint discomfort.

**8. Drugs and Medical treatments:** In rare circumstances, drugs or medical treatments may be required to properly control inflammation and joint discomfort. Healthcare providers frequently prescribe nonsteroidal anti-inflammatory medicines (NSAIDs), corticosteroids, and disease-modifying antirheumatic drugs (DMARDs) to decrease inflammation and relieve joint pain. Discuss these choices with your doctor to decide the best course of action for your unique problem.

## Enhanced Immune System Function

A healthy immune system is essential for safeguarding the body from dangerous microorganisms, infections, and illnesses. It works as a sophisticated network of cells, tissues, and organs to detect and destroy possible dangers. While the immune system is meant to defend the body, some lifestyle choices and behaviours can help to maintain and improve its performance. In this discussion, we will look at essential tactics for boosting and strengthening the immune system in order to achieve optimal health and well-being.

**1. A Nutrient-Rich and Balanced Diet:** A well-balanced diet rich in vital nutrients is needed for healthy immune system function. Consume a mix of fruits, vegetables, whole grains, lean proteins, healthy fats, and probiotic-rich foods. These contain vital vitamins (such as vitamin C, vitamin D, and zinc), minerals, antioxidants, and helpful microorganisms that help the immune system. Citrus fruits, berries, leafy greens, garlic, ginger, turmeric, yogurt, and fermented foods are excellent sources of immune-boosting nutrients.

**2. Adequate Hydration:** Keeping hydrated is critical for optimum immune function. Water aids in the movement of nutrients, the removal of contaminants, and the formation and flow of immune cells. Drink plenty of water throughout the day and think about introducing herbal teas, flavoured water, and other beverages, as well as hydrating items like cucumbers and watermelon, into your diet.

**3. Physical exercise on a Regular Basis:** Physical exercise on a regular basis is good for general health, including immune system function. Exercise improves blood circulation, allowing immune cells to circulate more efficiently throughout the body. Aim for at least 150 minutes per week of moderate-intensity aerobic activity as well as strength training activities to improve muscular strength and immunological response.

**4. Adequate Sleep:** Adequate sleep is essential for a healthy immune system. The body restores and regenerates during sleep, and the immune system releases essential cytokines that help control the immunological response. Aim for 7-9 hours of restful sleep every night and develop healthy sleep habits such as sticking to a consistent sleep schedule and creating a peaceful sleep environment.

**5. Stress Management:** Chronic stress can reduce immune function, making the body more susceptible to infections and disorders. To alleviate stress, use stress management practices such as meditation, deep breathing exercises, yoga, writing, or indulging in hobbies. Find relaxing hobbies and make time for self-care to help your immune system stay healthy.

**6. Avoid Smoking and Limit Alcohol use:** Smoking and excessive alcohol use can decrease immunological function and reduce the body's resistance against infections. To promote a healthy immune system, quit smoking if you are a smoker, and restrict alcohol consumption to moderate levels (up to one drink per day for women and two drinks per day for men).

**7. Good Hygiene Practices:** Regular handwashing with soap and water, correct coughing and sneezing etiquette, and keeping surfaces clean all assist in preventing the transmission of illnesses. These basic actions can protect you and others from viruses while also promoting a healthy immune system.

**8. Vaccinations:** Are essential for improving immune system function and avoiding particular illnesses. To improve your immune response against certain diseases, keep up with prescribed immunizations such as influenza, pneumonia, and other vaccines advised by healthcare providers.

# CHAPTER THREE

# UNDERSTANDING HIGH-LECTIN FOODS

## Common Foods High in Lectins

Lectins are plant-based proteins that may be found in a broad variety of foods. While lectins perform crucial functions in plants, such as insect control, they can be problematic for certain people owing to their tendency to induce digestive difficulties and other health issues. To make educated dietary decisions, it is critical to be aware of common foods high in lectins. In this detailed discussion, we will look at some of the most common foods that have high levels of lectins and analyse the possible consequences of eating them.

**1. Legumes:** Legumes, such as beans, lentils, chickpeas, and soybeans, are known to be high in lectins. The greatest lectin concentration is seen in raw or undercooked beans. Cooking processes like soaking, boiling, or fermenting, on the other hand, can drastically lower lectin levels and make them safer to ingest.

**2. Grains and Gluten-Containing Foods:** Certain grains, particularly those containing gluten, are high in lectins. Lectins are found in wheat, rye, barley, and goods manufactured from these grains, such as bread, pasta, and cereals. It is crucial to highlight, however, that the lectin concentration in properly cooked and processed grains is often lower and may not represent substantial hazards for the majority of people.

**3. Nightshade Vegetables:** Nightshade vegetables contain lectins, including tomatoes, potatoes, peppers (including bell peppers, chili peppers, and jalapenos), and eggplants. Cooking these veggies completely, on the other hand, can help lower lectin levels and make them more acceptable for people who are lectin-sensitive.

**4. Dairy products:** While dairy products are not often linked with high lectin content, some studies show that specific dairy proteins, such as casein and beta-lactoglobulin, may have lectin-like characteristics. However, lectin activity in dairy is usually thought to be minimal and not a major problem for most people.

**5. Seeds and Nuts:** Lectins are found in several seeds and nuts, including peanuts, cashews, sunflower seeds, and chia seeds. However, lectin concentrations in these foods are frequently lowered by suitable processing methods such as roasting or soaking. Most individuals tolerate these meals well, particularly when taken in moderation and properly cooked.

**6. Specific Fruits and Vegetables:** While most fruits and vegetables have low lectin concentrations, there are a few exceptions. Avocados and bananas, for example, contain lectins, although they are generally regarded as of minimal concern because most people tolerate them well. Berries, melons, and squashes are also lectin-rich fruits and vegetables, albeit in relatively modest quantities.

## The Hidden Sources of Lectins

Uncovering the Potential Culprits of Hidden Lectin Sources While certain foods are well-known for their lectin concentration, there are some lectin sources that may catch you off guard. These concealed sources can add to your overall lectin consumption and potentially harm your health, especially if you are lectin-sensitive. This talk will look at some of the hidden sources of lectins that you may come across in your regular life.

**1. Processed and Packaged Foods:** Many processed and packaged foods include lectin-rich components. Certain condiments, sauces, and dressings, for example, may contain tomato paste, which is rich in lectins. Modified food starch, soy protein isolate, and textured vegetable protein are also typical components to avoid since they can be obtained from lectin-containing sources. It is critical to carefully study ingredient labels and be aware of potential lectin sources in processed and packaged foods.

**2. Non-Food goods:** Lectins can be present in a variety of non-food goods, including supplements, pharmaceuticals, and personal care items. Some nutritional supplements, for example, may contain lectin-rich components such as legume-based protein powders or herbal extracts. It's critical to pay attention to the contents of these items, especially if you have lectin sensitivity or eat a low-lectin diet.

**3. Sprouted or Fermented Foods:** While sprouting and fermenting can help lower lectin concentrations in many foods, certain people who are extremely sensitive to lectins may still have negative effects. Sprouted or fermented foods such as sprouted grains, sprouted legumes, tempeh, and miso may contain residual lectins that might cause symptoms in people who are sensitive to them. It is critical to pay attention to your body and track your specific reaction to these foods.

**4. Cross-Infection:** When lectin-containing foods come into contact with other foods during storage, preparation, or cooking, cross-contamination can occur. If you cook lectin-containing beans in the same pot or use the same utensils without properly cleaning them, the lectins from the legumes may contaminate other meals. To avoid unintended lectin exposure, it is critical to practice excellent food hygiene and avoid cross-contamination.

**5. Hidden substances:** Although certain substances are not obvious sources of lectins, they might nonetheless contain lectin activity. Flavors enhancers such as monosodium glutamate (MSG) and hydrolysed vegetable protein (HVP), for example, can be obtained from lectin-rich sources and may contribute to your total lectin consumption. When making dietary choices, be mindful of these hidden substances and their possible lectin levels.

**6. Sprayed or Treated Produce:** Some commercially produced fruits and vegetables may have been sprayed or treated with lectin-inducing chemicals. In traditional agriculture, pesticides, herbicides, and fungicides may introduce lectins into the crop. Choosing organic or locally grown vegetables can help decrease your exposure to lectin-rich compounds.

### Identifying Lectin Content in Foods

It is critical to have the information and skills to determine the lectin content in the foods you consume while following a low-lectin diet or attempting to decrease lectin exposure. While determining the exact lectin levels in individual foods might be difficult, there are various ways you can use to make better educated decisions. In this detailed discussion, we will look at numerous methods and factors to consider when determining lectin concentration in food.

**1. Research and Reference:** Begin by learning about common foods that are strong in lectins. Learn about the lectin composition of several dietary categories, such as legumes, grains, nightshade vegetables, and seeds. Look for credible sources, scientific studies, and books written by lectin and nutrition experts. These tools can help you make educated decisions by providing vital information regarding the lectin content of certain foods.

**2. Cooking and Processing procedures:** Cooking and processing procedures can have a substantial impact on the lectin content in foods. Soaking, boiling, fermenting, and pressure cooking are some cooking methods that might help lower lectin levels. Soaking beans overnight and then fully boiling them, for example, can considerably reduce lectin levels. Similarly, fermenting foods such as cabbage into sauerkraut or creating sourdough bread from fermented grains can help to reduce lectin levels. Understanding the effect of different cooking and processing methods on lectin levels might help you make better food preparation decisions.

**3. Individual Tolerance and Sensitivity:** It is critical to understand that individual tolerance to lectins varies greatly. Some people are more sensitive to lectins and may have negative effects even at low amounts, whilst others may tolerate larger levels with no problems. Keep track of your body's reactions to different foods and any symptoms or changes in your overall health. Keeping a food journal can help you find potential links between particular foods and symptoms, which can help you make better decisions.

**4. customised Testing:** Individuals with suspected lectin sensitivity or specific health issues may be eligible for customised testing. These tests can offer information on lectin reactivity or immunological responses in individuals. It is important to seek the advice of a healthcare practitioner or a trained dietician who specializes in lectin-related issues can assess the applicability and reliability of such testing for your unique need.

**5. Label Reading:** When purchasing packaged and processed goods, it is critical to read the ingredient labels. Look for items that are high in lectins, such as legumes, grains, and nightshade vegetables. Soy, wheat, corn, and tomato-based components are common examples. Be aware that certain concealed sources of lectins may have several names, so get familiar with the many names or words that may signal the existence of lectins.

# CHAPTER FOUR

# GETTING STARTED: TRANSITIONING TO A LOW LECTIN DIET

## Preparing Your Mindset for Change

Starting a new dietary strategy, such as a reduced-lectin diet, necessitates not just nutritional modifications but also a mental shift. Adopting a positive and open mentality can help smooth the adjustment and boost your chances of long-term success.

**1. Educate Yourself:** Begin by learning about lectins and their possible influence on health. Learn about the science of lectins, their origins, and how they might influence your health. As you begin your new nutritional adventure, this information will equip you to make educated decisions and provide you with a sense of purpose and direction.

**2.Set Clear Goal:** Define your goals and motivations for following a low-lectin diet. Are you looking for relief from specific health conditions, more energy, or to enhance your general well-being? Having clear and defined goals will provide you with a sense of purpose and the desire to stick to your dietary modifications.

**3. Adopt a Growth mentality:** Develop a growth mentality by believing in your potential to change and viewing setbacks as opportunities for learning and progress. Understand that switching to a low-lectin diet may require modifications, experimenting, and learning from your mistakes. Accept the perspective that setbacks are transient and that, with dedication and tenacity, you can overcome them.

**4. Pay Attention to the Benefits:** Pay attention to the possible benefits of a reduced lectin diet. Remind yourself of the benefits you expect, such as better digestion, less inflammation, more energy, and general well-being. Consider how these advantages will improve your quality of life and act as a source of inspiration through difficult times.

**5. Practice Self-Compassion:** Be kind with yourself during the transition period. Recognize that change takes time and that it is natural to meet roadblocks along the way. Avoid self-judgment or feelings of guilt if you mess up or find it difficult to stick to the dietary modifications at first. Instead, be compassionate to yourself, forgive yourself, and view setbacks as chances to learn and develop.

**6. Seek Help:** Seek help from loved ones, friends, or online groups who have similar nutritional objectives. Having a support structure along the way may give encouragement, accountability, and a sense of belonging. Share your experiences, get guidance, and rejoice in your accomplishments together. Consider working with a certified dietician or a healthcare practitioner who can give tailored advice and assistance.

**7. Develop a Mindful Eating Practice:** Develop a mindful eating practice by paying attention to the present moment when eating. Slow down, taste your food's aromas and textures, and be totally present with each bite. Mindful eating allows you to become more aware of your body's hunger and fullness cues, develops a healthy connection with food, and improves your entire eating experience.

**8. Value Variety and Experimentation:** Approach your low-lectin diet with curiosity and an open mind. Accept the opportunity to try new cuisines, tastes, and recipes. Experiment with various cooking methods, spices, and seasonings to improve the Flavors and enjoyment of your meals. Embracing diversity and culinary innovation can help make the nutritional adjustment more fun and lasting

**9. Recognize and appreciate success:** Recognize and appreciate your success along the journey, no matter how minor it may appear. Recognize your efforts in making beneficial dietary adjustments as well as the milestones you reach. Reward yourself with non-food delights, such as self-care activities, relaxing techniques, or engaging in hobbies that you like.

## Pantry Makeover: Eliminating High-Lectin Foods

One of the most important steps in starting a low-lectin diet is a pantry makeover. Selecting your pantry lectin-free lays the groundwork for selecting healthier food choices and supporting your nutritional objectives. Here, we'll go over the methods for removing high-lectin goods from your pantry as well as practical advice for a successful pantry makeover.

**1. Take Stock:** Begin by taking stock of the goods in your pantry. This entails looking over each shelf and finding lectin-rich items. Legumes (such as beans, lentils, and chickpeas), grains (such as wheat, barley, and rye), nightshade vegetables (such as tomatoes, peppers, and eggplants), and some seeds (such as chia seeds and pumpkin seeds) are examples of high-lectin meals.

**2. Read Labels:** Inspect the labels of packaged and processed items in your cupboard. Look for substances produced from high-lectin sources, as these might appear in a variety of ways. Ingredients such as soy, maize, wheat flour, and tomato-based products are examples of probable lectin-containing ingredients. Keep in mind that certain goods may have several labels for high-lectin components, so become aware of the many terms that may signal their existence.

**3. Remove High-Lectin items:** Once you've found the high-lectin items in your cupboard, get rid of them. Items that no longer fit your low-lectin diet goals should be discarded or donated. By removing these items, you make physical and mental room for the addition of low-lectin alternatives that promote your health.

**4. Stock up on Low-Lectin Substitutes:**

To ensure you have healthy options on hand, replace high-lectin foods with low-lectin ones. Include a range of fresh vegetables (excluding nightshades), low-sugar fruits, healthy fats (such as avocados and olive oil), lean proteins (such as chicken, fish, and grass-fed meats), and gluten-free grains (such as quinoa and rice). It's also a good idea to keep a variety of herbs, spices, and condiments on hand to boost the Flavors of your dishes.

**5. Organize and Arrange:** Reorganize your pantry so that low-lectin goods are easy to find. Similar commodities, such as cereals, nuts and seeds, oils, and canned foods, should be grouped together. Consider storing bulk materials in transparent containers or jars and labelling them for ease. A well-organized pantry not only makes it easier to discover items, but it also fosters a sense of order and control over your food choices.

**6. Make a Shopping List:** Make a list of low-lectin goods and items that you'll need to have a well-rounded, healthy pantry. To ensure you achieve your nutritional needs, plan your meals ahead of time and include a variety of components. A thorough shopping list can make supermarket excursions more effective and will assist you in sticking to your low-lectin diet.

**7. Be Aware of Cross-Contamination:** Be aware of the possibility of cross-contamination of high-lectin goods in your pantry. Make sure that flours, grains, and legumes are properly wrapped to avoid inadvertent contamination with other foods. This is especially critical if you have family members who continue to eat high-lectin foods. Consider separating storage spaces or using containers with clearly labelled lids to reduce the possibility of cross-contamination.

**8. Educate home Members:** If you share your pantry with other members of your home who may continue to eat high-lectin items, it is critical that you educate them about your dietary objectives and the need to keep high-lectin and low-lectin goods separate.

Separate the little things. A peaceful pantry environment may be maintained through clear communication and mutual respect for each other's dietary preferences.

**9. Seek Help:** Transitioning to a reduced lectin diet can be difficult, so don't be afraid to seek help from loved ones, friends, or online forums. Share your pantry makeover adventure with others who follow a similar nutritional approach and exchange ideas, recipes, and advice. Their advice and shared experiences might be beneficial as you make this nutritional transition.

## Grocery Shopping Guide: Selecting Low Lectin Foods

Making prudent grocery store decisions is critical when following a low-lectin diet. You can promote your health and well-being while enjoying a range of nutritional alternatives by eating foods low in lectins. Here is a detailed grocery shopping guide to help you choose low-lectin foods:

**1. Fresh veggies:** Choose non-starchy veggies that are low in lectins. Choose leafy greens like spinach, kale, and arugula over cruciferous veggies like broccoli, cauliflower, and Brussels sprouts. Zucchini, cucumber, asparagus, green beans, and mushrooms are also low in lectins. Avoid nightshade vegetables such as tomatoes, peppers, and eggplants since they contain greater quantities of lectins.

**2. Fruits with Low Sugar Content:** Choose fruits with minimal sugar and lectin levels. Strawberries, blueberries, and raspberries are all wonderful choices. Apples, pears, and cherries have minimal lectin content and can be consumed in moderation. However, high-sugar foods such as bananas, grapes, and melons should be limited or avoided.

**3. Lean Proteins:** Choose lean protein sources that are low in lectins. Poultry such as chicken and turkey, wild-caught fish such as salmon and cod, and eggs are examples. In moderation, grass-fed beef and lamb are also good alternatives. Plant-based proteins like tofu, tempeh, and fermented soy products can be included provided you tolerate them well; however, some people are sensitive to soy lectins.

**4. Storage Low-Lectin Substitutes:** To ensure you have healthy options on hand, replace high-lectin foods with low-lectin ones. Include a range of fresh vegetables (excluding nightshades), low-sugar fruits, healthy fats (such as avocados and olive oil), lean proteins (such as chicken, fish, and grass-fed meats), and gluten-free grains (such as quinoa and rice). It's also a good idea to keep a variety of herbs, spices, and condiments on hand to boost the flavor of your dishes.

**5. Organize and rearrange:** your cupboard to make low-lectin goods more accessible. Similar commodities, such as cereals, nuts and seeds, oils, and canned foods, should be grouped together. Consider storing bulk materials in transparent containers or jars and labeling them for ease. An organized pantry not only makes finding items easier, but it also creates a sense of order and gives you control over your nutritional choices.

**6. Herbs and spices:** Use a variety of herbs and spices to enhance the taste of your dishes. Many herbs and spices, including basil, oregano, thyme, rosemary, turmeric, and ginger, are low in lectins and contribute flavor as well as health benefits to your meals.

**7. Dairy substitutes:** Choose unsweetened and unflavored dairy substitutes such as almond milk, coconut milk, or oat milk if you want to consume dairy alternatives. These plant-based milk substitutes often contain less lectin than regular dairy products.

**8. Legume Substitutes:** Because legumes are high in lectins, look for substitutes that have similar nutritional advantages. Consider adding lentils, which have lower lectin levels than other legumes, or non-legume choices such as chickpea pasta or bean-free hummus.

**9. Fermented Foods:** Fermented foods can contain helpful probiotics and enzymes, so include these on your shopping list. Consider sauerkraut, kimchi, coconut yogurt, and kombucha. Fermentation can help lower the amount of lectins in some foods, making them more acceptable for some people.

**10. Organic and Locally produced Foods:** Choose organic and locally produced fruit and meats wherever feasible. Organic foods are typically devoid of synthetic pesticides and chemicals, whereas locally produced foods are frequently fresher and more nutrient-dense.

# CHAPTER FIVE

# THE LOW LECTIN DIET PLAN

## Creating Balanced and Nutritious Meals

While following a low-lectin diet, it is essential to prepare balanced and nutritious meals to support your overall health and well-being. Here are some pointers to help you create a balanced and fulfilling meal plan:

**1. Eat a Variety of Non-Starchy Vegetables:** Non-starchy vegetables should form the basis of your meals. They are high in vitamins, minerals, and fiber but low in lectins. Colorful vegetables such as leafy greens, broccoli, cauliflower, asparagus, and green beans should account for at least half of your meal. These veggies not only supply essential nutrients, but they also add bulk and texture to your dishes.

**2. Include Lean Proteins:** Choose lean protein sources to help with muscle development and repair. Choose skinless poultry, fish, seafood, tofu, tempeh, and eggs. These protein sources are lectin-free and include necessary amino acids. Keep portion sizes in mind and balance your meal with a suitable quantity of protein.

**3. Incorporate Healthy Fats:** Include healthy fats in your meals to increase satiety and support numerous biological processes. Healthy fats may be found in avocados, olive oil, coconut oil, nuts, and seeds. These ingredients enhance the flavor and texture of your meals. Remember that fats are high in calories, so eat them in moderation.

**4. Select Gluten-Free Grains and Pseudocereals:** If you handle grains well, select gluten-free choices like quinoa, rice (both white and brown), and gluten-free oats. These grains have few lectins and can supply important minerals and fiber. Pseudocereals such as amaranth and buckwheat can also be used as nutritional substitutes.

**5. Don't Forget Legume Substitutes:** Because conventional legumes are heavy in lectins, look for legume substitutes that can give similar advantages. Lentils, for example, have a reduced lectin content and can be used in soups, stews, and salads. Another alternative is chickpea pasta, which is prepared from ground chickpeas. These legume substitutes provide plant-based protein and fiber while reducing lectin exposure.

**6. Highlight Herbs and Spices:** Instead of depending on high-lectin condiments and sauces, use herbs and spices to enhance the flavor of your food. Herbs and spices like basil, oregano, turmeric, cinnamon, and garlic powder may add depth and variety to your foods while avoiding the introduction of lectins.

**7. Eat Fiber-Rich Foods First:** Fiber is essential for digestive health and maintaining normal blood sugar levels. Include fiber-rich foods such as nonstarchy vegetables, fruits (in moderation), whole grains (if tolerated), and chia seeds in your diet. These foods help with digestion, satiety, and general gut health.

**8. Hydrate with Water:** Water is necessary for adequate hydration and aids in the maintenance of optimal body functioning. Make water your primary beverage of choice, and minimize your intake of sugary beverages and artificial sweeteners. Hydration is essential for digestion, vitamin absorption, and general health.

**9. Plan and Prep Ahead:** To ensure you have nutritious meals on hand, plan and prepare your meals ahead of time. Make time to plan meals, make a shopping list, and prepare ingredients. Batch cooking and portioning foods can help you save time and stay on track with your low-lectin diet throughout the week.

**10. Seek ideas and Variety:** For recipe ideas, go through recipe books, online resources, and low-lectin-friendly forums. Variety is essential for receiving a diverse variety of nutrients and avoiding dietary monotony. Experiment with new tastes, cooking methods, and ingredients to keep your meals fresh and intriguing.

**Sample Meal Plans for Breakfast, Lunch, and Dinner**

**Sample Breakfast Meal Plan:**

**Option 1: Veggie Omelet**

**Ingredients:**

- Eggs
- Spinach
- Mushrooms
- Onions

**Instructions:** Beat eggs, sauté spinach, mushrooms, and onions. Pour the beaten eggs over the cooked veggies and cook until the omelet is set. Serve with sliced avocado on the side.

**Option 2: Chia Seed Pudding**

**Ingredients:**

- Chia seeds
- Unsweetened almond milk
- Berries
- Nuts

**Instructions:** Mix chia seeds with almond milk and refrigerate overnight. In the morning, add fresh berries and a sprinkle of nuts for crunch.

**Sample Lunch Meal Plan:**

**Option 1: Grilled Chicken Salad**

**Ingredients:**

- Grilled chicken breast
- mixed greens
- cucumber
- cherry tomatoes
- avocado
- olive oil
- lemon juice

**Instructions:** Combine greens, cucumber, tomatoes, and avocado. Top with grilled chicken breast. Drizzle with olive oil and lemon juice.

**Option 2: Quinoa and Vegetable Stir-Fry**

**Ingredients:**

- Quinoa
- Mixed stir-fry vegetables (broccoli, bell peppers, snap peas)
- Tofu or shrimp

- Tamari sauce
- Sesame oil

**Instructions:**

Cook quinoa as directed. In a separate pan, stir-fry mixed vegetables and protein with tamari sauce and sesame oil. Serve over quinoa.

Sample Dinner Meal Plan:

**Option 1: Baked Salmon with Roasted Vegetables**
**Ingredients:**

- Salmon fillet
- Asparagus
- Bell peppers
- Red onion
- Olive oil
- Lemon
- Fresh herbs (such as dill or parsley)

**Instructions:**

Place salmon on a baking sheet. Top with lemon juice, olive oil, and herbs. Roast until cooked through. Toss asparagus, bell peppers, and red onion with oil and roast until tender. Serve salmon with roasted vegetables.

**Option 2: Zucchini Noodles with Turkey Bolognese**

**Ingredients:**

- Zucchini
- Ground turkey
- Diced tomatoes
- Tomato paste
- Onion
- Garlic
- Italian seasoning
- Olive oil

**Instructions:**

Spiralize zucchini into noodles. In a separate pan, cook ground turkey with diced onion and garlic until browned. Add tomatoes, tomato paste, and Italian seasoning. Simmer until flavors meld. Serve Bolognese sauce over zucchini noodles.

## Snack Ideas and Healthy Alternatives

Snack time is an opportunity to fuel your body with nutritious options that keep you satisfied between meals. Here are some snack ideas and healthy alternatives to consider:

**1.FreshFruit:**

Enjoy a variety of fresh fruits like berries, sliced apples, oranges, or grapes. They provide natural sweetness, fiber, and essential vitamins.

**2.Vegetable Sticks with Hummus:** Slice up crunchy vegetables such as carrot sticks, cucumber rounds, or bell pepper strips. Pair them with a serving of hummus for a satisfying and nutrient-rich snack.

**3.Nuts and Seeds:** Grab a handful of unsalted almonds, walnuts, or pumpkin seeds. They are packed with healthy fats, protein, and fiber, providing sustained energy and satiety.

**4. Greek Yogurt with Berries:**Choose plain Greek yogurt and top it with a handful of fresh berries for a protein-rich and antioxidant-packed snack. Add a drizzle of honey or a sprinkle of cinnamon for extra flavor.

**5. Rice Cakes with Nut Butter:** Opt for whole-grain rice cakes and spread them with a tablespoon of almond butter, peanut butter, or sunflower seed butter. It's a satisfying combination of crunch and creaminess.

**6. Hard-Boiled Eggs:**Hard-boiled eggs are a convenient and protein-rich snack option. Sprinkle them with a pinch of salt and pepper, or enjoy them with a side of sliced vegetables.

**7. Roasted Chickpeas:** Make your own roasted chickpeas by tossing cooked chickpeas with olive oil and spices like paprika, cumin, or garlic powder. Roast them in the oven until crispy for a flavorful and fiber-rich snack.

**8. Dark Chocolate:** Indulge in a square or two of dark chocolate with a high cocoa content (70% or higher). It's a delicious way to satisfy your sweet tooth while benefiting from antioxidants.

**9. Homemade Trail Mix:** Create your own trail mix by combining a mix of unsalted nuts, dried fruits, and seeds. Customize it with your favorite combinations for a portable and nutritious snack.

**10.Veggie Wraps:** Wrap fresh vegetables like lettuce, cucumber, bell peppers, and avocado in a large lettuce leaf or collard green leaf. Add a protein source such as turkey slices or tofu for a refreshing and low-carb snack.

## Adapting the Low Lectin Diet to Different Lifestyles (e.g., vegetarian, vegan)

The Low Lectin Diet can be customized to accommodate various dietary preferences and lifestyles, including vegetarian and vegan approaches. While the diet emphasizes reducing high-lectin foods, it does not necessarily require the complete elimination of all plant-based foods. Here are some tips for adapting the low-lecithin diet to vegetarian and vegan lifestyles:

1. **Vegetarian Adaptation:** For those following a vegetarian diet, the focus is on eliminating high-lectin animal products while still incorporating a variety of plant-based foods. Here are some guidelines:

- **Protein Sources:** Include plant-based protein sources such as legumes (lentils, chickpeas, and black beans), tofu, tempeh, edamame, and plant-based protein powders. These options provide essential amino acids without the high lectin content found in certain animal proteins.

- **Nuts and Seeds:** Incorporate a variety of nuts and seeds like almonds, walnuts, chia seeds, and flaxseeds. They offer healthy fats, protein, and fiber while being low in lectins.

- **Dairy Alternatives:** If you consume dairy, opt for low-lactose options like lactose-free milk or yogurt and cheese made from non-dairy sources like almond, cashew, or coconut.

- **Whole Grains:** Choose gluten-free whole grains like quinoa, brown rice, millet, and buckwheat. These grains are low in lectins and provide essential nutrients and fiber.

**2. Vegan Adaptation:** A vegan diet excludes all animal products, including meat, dairy, eggs, and honey. Here's how to adapt the low-lecithin diet to a vegan lifestyle:

- **Legumes as Protein:** Rely on a variety of legumes like lentils, chickpeas, black beans, and soybeans as primary protein sources. Legumes are low in lectins when properly prepared by soaking and cooking.

- **Plant-Based Milk and Alternatives:** Substitute dairy milk with plant-based alternatives like almond milk, coconut milk, or oat milk. Choose unsweetened options to minimize added sugars.

- **Nutritional Yeast:** Nutritional yeast can be used as a flavorful, vegan-friendly substitute for cheese. It adds a cheesy, nutty taste to dishes and is a good source of B vitamins.

- **Healthy Fats:** Include sources of healthy fats in your diet, such as
- Avocados

- Nuts

- Seeds

- and plant-based oils like

- Olive oil

- Avocado oil or coconut oil.

**Seaweed and Algae:** Incorporate seaweed and algae, such as nori, wakame, or spirulina, into your diet to ensure adequate intake of essential minerals and omega-3 fatty acids.

# CHAPTER SIX

# COOKING TECHNIQUES AND RECIPES

## Cooking Methods that Reduce Lectin Content

When following a low lectin diet, it is critical to use cooking methods that lower the lectin content of foods. You may reduce the amount of lectins in particular substances by utilizing specialized strategies. Here are several culinary methods that might assist you in accomplishing this:

**1. Soaking:** Soaking beans, grains, and seeds before cooking can help reduce lectin levels. Soaking the lectins for several hours or overnight causes them to leach into the water. Discarding the soaking water and cooking with fresh water may further lower the lectin concentration.

**2.Sprouting:** Sprouting legumes, grains, and seeds is another excellent strategy to reduce lectins. Sprouting is the process of soaking seeds until they germinate and begin to sprout. Not only does this technique lower lectin levels, but it also increases nutrient availability and digestion.

**3. Boiling:** Foods can be reduced in lectin concentration by boiling them. You may efficiently reduce lectin levels by cooking beans, grains, and some vegetables in boiling water. To eradicate any leftover lectins, vigorous cooking is required.

**4. Pressure Cooking:** Using a pressure cooker to minimize lectin concentration in meals is an effective method. The intense heat and pressure created during pressure cooking can efficiently break down lectins. This approach is especially beneficial for legumes with high lectin content, such as beans.

**5. Fermentation:** Certain foods can be greatly reduced in lectin concentration by fermenting them. Beneficial bacteria that can break down lectins proliferate during fermentation. Fermented veggies, tempeh, and miso are low in lectins and high in probiotics, which promote gut health.

**6. Peeling and Removing Seeds:** Lectins can be concentrated in the skin or seeds of particular fruits and vegetables. Lectin consumption can be reduced by peeling and removing the seeds. To remove the skin and seeds off tomatoes, cucumbers, and squash, for example.

**7. High-Heat Cooking:** High-temperature grilling, broiling, and roasting can help break down lectins. These procedures subject foods to high heat, which reduces lectin levels. However, excessive charring or burning should be avoided since it might produce potentially hazardous chemicals.

**8. Combination Cooking:** Combining different cooking methods can also help reduce lectin levels. To further reduce lectin levels, soak legumes first, then pressure cook them, and then utilize high-heat cooking methods like grilling or roasting.

## Delicious Low Lectin Recipes for Every Occasion

A lectin-free diet does not entail compromising flavor or diversity. You can cook healthy and tasty meals with a little imagination and the correct components. Here are some delectable low-lectin dishes for various occasions.

**1.Breakfast:**

Spinach and Mushroom Frittata:

**Ingredients:**

- 4 large eggs
- 1 cup spinach, chopped
- 1 cup mushrooms, sliced
- 1\2 cup onions, diced
- Salt and pepper to taste
- 1 tablespoon olive oil

**Instructions for Spinach and Mushroom Omelet with Avocado:**

**1.** Beat the eggs in a bowl and season with salt and pepper.

**2.** Heat olive oil in a non-stick skillet over medium heat.

**3.** Sauté spinach, mushrooms, and onions until softened.

**4.** Pour the beaten eggs over the cooked veggies.

**5.** Cook until the omelet is set.

**6.** Serve with a side of sliced avocado.

**2. Lunch:**

**Greek Salad with Grilled Chicken:**

**Ingredients:**

- 2 cups mixed greens
- 1/2 cucumber sliced
- 1/2 cup cherry tomatoes
- halved1/2 avocado, diced
- 4 oz. grilled chicken breast, sliced
- 1 tablespoon olive oil
- Juice of 1/2 lemon
- Salt and pepper to taste

**Instructions:**

**1.** Combine mixed greens, cucumber, cherry tomatoes, and avocado in a large bowl.

**2.** Add grilled chicken breast slices on top.

**3.** Drizzle with olive oil and lemon juice.

**4.** Season with salt and pepper.

**5.** Gently toss to combine and savor a revitalizing and nourishing salad.

**3. Dinner:** Zucchini Noodles with Pesto Sauce

**Ingredients:**

- 2 medium zucchini, spiralized
- 1/2 cup fresh basil leaves
- 1/4 cup pine nuts
- 2 cloves of garlic
- 3 tablespoons of olive oil
- Juice of 1/2 lemon
- Salt and pepper to taste

**Instructions:**

**1.** Combine basil leaves, pine nuts, garlic, olive oil, lemon juice, salt, and pepper in a food processor.

**2.** Process until smooth, creating a flavorful pesto sauce.

**3.** Heat olive oil in a large skillet over medium heat.

**4.** Add zucchini noodles and sauté until tender, for a few minutes.

**5.** Stir in the pesto sauce and gently toss to coat the noodles.

**6.** Serve the dish hot, garnishing with extra basil leaves if desired.

## 4. Snack:

- **Roasted Chickpeas:**

**Ingredients:**

- 1 can (15 oz) chickpeas, drained and rinsed
- 1 tablespoon olive oil
- 1 teaspoon paprika
- 1/2 teaspoon cumin
- 1/2 teaspoon garlic powder
- Salt to taste

**Instructions:**

1. Preheat the oven to 400°F (200°C).

2. Pat the chickpeas dry to remove excess moisture.

3. In a bowl, combine chickpeas, olive oil, paprika, cumin, garlic powder, and salt.

4. Spread the chickpeas in a single layer on a baking sheet.

5. Roast in the oven for 20–25 minutes until crispy and golden brown.

6. Remove from the oven and let cool before enjoying a crunchy and healthy snack.

**5. Dessert:**

- **Berry Chia Seed Pudding:**

**Ingredients:**

- 1/4 cup chia seeds
- 1 cup unsweetened almond milk
- 1 tablespoon maple syrup
- 1/2 teaspoons of vanilla extract
- Fresh berries for topping

**Instructions:**

1. Combine chia seeds, almond milk, maple syrup, and vanilla extract in a bowl.

2. Stir thoroughly to ensure an even distribution of chia seeds.

3. Allow the mixture to sit for 10 minutes, stirring again to prevent clumping.

4. Cover the bowl and refrigerate for a minimum of 4 hours or overnight, allowing the chia seeds to absorb the liquid and create a pudding-like consistency.

5. Prior to serving, garnish with fresh berries to enhance sweetness and introduce a burst of flavor.

## Recipe Modifications and Ingredient Substitutions

You may need to alter a recipe to meet your dietary requirements, tastes, or ingredient availability. With a little imagination, you can make changes and substitutions while retaining the general flavor of the dish. Here are some suggestions for recipe changes and ingredient substitutions:

**1. Flour Substitutions:** For gluten-free recipes, use almond flour, coconut flour, or gluten-free flour blends for all-purpose flour.

- Consider using whole wheat flour or a combination of whole wheat and all-purpose flour to make dishes more healthy.

**2. Sugar Substitutions:**

- Use natural sweeteners like honey, maple syrup, or agave nectar instead of refined sugar.

- For a lower glycemic index option, try using stevia or monk fruit sweetener.

## 3. Dairy Substitutions:

- Replace cow's milk with almond milk, coconut milk, oat milk, or soy milk for a dairy-free alternative.
- Swap butter with plant-based oils like olive oil or coconut oil.

**4. Egg Substitutions:** Replace eggs in baking recipes with applesauce, mashed bananas, or yogurt.

- Tofu, flaxseed meal, or chickpea flour combined with water can be used in savory meals.

**5. Meat Substitutions:** For vegetarian or vegan meals, use plant-based protein sources like tofu, tempeh, or legumes like lentils or beans instead of meat.

- To lower saturated fat levels, use leaner cuts of meat or poultry.

**6. Seasoning Changes:** Depending on your taste, adjust the amount of salt, herbs, and spices.

- Experiment with various herbs and spices to bring distinct tastes to the meal.

**7. Vegetable Substitutions:** If a recipe specifies a certain vegetable, feel free to use a comparable one that you like or have on hand.

- You may also boost the nutritional content of the dish by adding more veggies.

**8. Allergy-Friendly Modifications:** When making recipe changes, keep allergens like nuts, gluten,or dairy in mind. Look for acceptable substitutes or leave out the allergenic substances completely.

# CHAPTER SEVEN

# SUPPLEMENTING YOUR LOW LECTIN DIET

## Key Nutrients to Support Health on a Low Lectin Diet

When following a low-lectin diet, it is critical to ensure that you are still getting essential nutrients to support overall health and well-being. Here are some key nutrients to consider when planning your meals on a low-lectin diet:

**1. Protein:**

Include adequate protein sources to support muscle growth, repair, and overall health. Choose lean sources of animal protein such as poultry, fish, and eggs or plant-based options such as legumes, tofu, tempeh, and quinoa.

**2. Healthy Fats:** Add healthy fats to your diet to help with brain function, hormone synthesis, and nutrition absorption. Avocados, almonds, seeds, olive oil, coconut oil, and fatty seafood like salmon are all good sources of healthy fats. These fats also aid in enhancing satiety and offer energy.

## 3. Fiber:

Consume fiber-rich meals to improve digestive health, control blood sugar levels, and produce a sense of fullness. Dietary fiber is abundant in non-starchy vegetables, fruits in moderation, whole grains (if tolerated), nuts, and seeds. Consume a variety of these meals to get different kinds of fiber.

## 4. Vitamins and Minerals:

Eat a variety of fruits and vegetables to ensure proper vitamin and mineral consumption. Vitamins A, C, and K, as well as minerals like iron, calcium, and magnesium, are abundant in dark leafy greens, colorful berries, cruciferous vegetables, and citrus fruits. If required, consider supplementing.

## 5. Omega-3 Fatty Acids:

Include omega-3 fatty acids in your diet to improve heart health, cognitive function, and inflammation reduction. Omega-3s are abundant in fatty fish such as salmon, mackerel, and sardines. Flaxseeds, chia seeds, and walnuts are examples of plant-based sources. If your nutritional consumption is insufficient, consider taking omega-3 supplements.

## 6. Antioxidants:

Consume antioxidant-rich foods to help counteract oxidative stress and inflammation. Antioxidants are abundant in berries, dark chocolate, green tea, colorful vegetables, and herbs such as turmeric and ginger. These substances serve to protect cells and promote general health.

**7. Calcium and Vitamin D:** Maintain enough calcium and vitamin D consumption to maintain bone health. Include calcium- and vitamin D-enriched dairy or dairy substitutes, leafy greens like kale and broccoli, and fortified plant-based milk replacements. Spend time outside to increase natural vitamin D production.

**8. Hydration:** Don't overlook the necessity of being hydrated. Consume enough water throughout the day to aid digestion, nutritional absorption, and general body processes. Aim for at least 8 cups. (64 ounces) of water each day, and modify as needed based on activity level and individual needs.

### Recommended Supplements and their Benefits

While it is usually preferable to get nutrients from whole foods, some people may benefit from supplements to augment their low-lectin diet. Here are several supplements that have been recommended and their potential benefits:

**1. Omega-3 Fatty Acids:** Omega-3 supplements such as fish oil or algae-based supplements include important fatty acids such as EPA and DHA. They promote heart health, cognitive function, and inflammation reduction. Omega-3 supplements are especially advantageous for people who do not consume fatty fish on a daily basis.

**2. Vitamin D:** Vitamin D is important for bone health, immunological function, and mood management. Because it can be difficult to receive enough vitamin D from diet alone, especially for individuals who get little sun, a vitamin D supplement may be advantageous. To find the optimum dose for your needs, it is essential to check with a healthcare expert.

**3. Probiotics:** Probiotic pills include helpful microorganisms that aid in the maintenance of a healthy gut flora. They can help with digestion, immunological function, and general gut health. For best efficacy, look for a high-quality probiotic supplement that contains many types of bacteria.

**4. Multivitamin and Mineral Supplement:** A multivitamin and mineral supplement can help address nutritional deficiencies in your diet. Look for a supplement that contains B vitamins, vitamin C, vitamin E,

magnesium, zinc, and selenium, among other things. Choose a renowned brand and get tailored advice from a healthcare practitioner.

**5. Digestive Enzymes:** Digestive enzyme supplements can help with nutrition breakdown and absorption. They may be useful for those who have digestive disorders or who have trouble digesting particular foods. Look for an enzyme combination that contains protease, amylase, and lipase.

**6. Antioxidants:**

Supplementing with antioxidants such as vitamin C, vitamin E, and selenium can help neutralize harmful free radicals and reduce oxidative stress. Antioxidants support overall cellular health and may provide benefits for skin health, immune function, and aging.

# CHAPTER EIGHT

# OVERCOMING CHALLENGES AND MAINTAINING LONG-TERM SUCCESS

## Strategies for Dining Out on a Low Lectin Diet

Dining out while on a low-lectin diet might be difficult, but with a little planning and strategy, you can navigate restaurant menus and find choices that meet your dietary needs. Here are some tips for eating out on a low-lectin diet:

**1. Research and Plan Ahead:** Before visiting a restaurant, spend some time researching their menu online. Look for recipes that are low in lectins or that can be readily changed. Many restaurants now provide thorough menus, including ingredient listings, to assist you in making educated decisions.

**2. Select Simple Preparations:** Choose foods that are prepared simply, such as grilled, steamed, or roasted. These approaches are less likely to employ high-lectin cooking procedures or excessively added additives. To limit the danger of hidden lectin sources, request that your meal be cooked without sauces, marinades, or breading.

**3. Personalize Your purchase:** Don't be hesitant to ask questions and make changes to your purchase. Most establishments are ready to accommodate special dietary requirements. Request high-lectin food swaps or omissions, such as substituting grains for more veggies or replacing sauces with olive oil and lemon juice.

**4. Prioritize Vegetables and Protein:** When planning your meal, prioritize vegetable-based meals and lean protein selections. Salads, grilled veggies, and grilled or baked meats or fish are also good options. Make sure the veggies are prepared in a lectin-free manner and that the protein is not overly marinated or breaded.

**5. Be Wary of Hidden Sources:** Be wary of hidden lectin sources such as sauces, dressings, and condiments. Request that these be served on the side or eliminated entirely. Soups, stews, and casseroles should be avoided since they may include high-lectin items such as legumes or nightshade vegetables.

**6. Communicate with the Staff:** Inform your server of your dietary limitations and request their assistance. They may be able to recommend lectin-free alternatives or offer information on component composition. Clear communication can help guarantee that your requirements are understood and treated correctly.

**7. Selecting Ethnic Cuisines Wisely:**

Certain ethnic foods have a lower lectin content. Mediterranean, Japanese, and seafood-focused restaurants, for example, frequently provide meals that are compatible with a low-lectin diet. Menus include grilled fish, seaweed, salads, and vegetable-based items to try.

**8. Concentrate on Your Overall Meal Plan:** If your restaurant of choice does not have many low-lectin alternatives, try altering your daily meal plan. Consume a lighter dinner or snack before heading out to give yourself more options. You may also prepare ahead of time by choosing low-lectin foods for other meals throughout the day.

### Navigating Social Situations and Family Gatherings

Navigating social events and family gatherings while on a low-lectin diet may require some extra forethought and communication. Here are some tips to help you effectively manage these situations:

**1. Plan Ahead:**

Inform the host or organizer of your dietary needs before

attending social events or family gatherings. Inform them of your low-lectin diet and ask if they can accommodate your needs or if you can bring food that meets your dietary restrictions.

## 2. Offer to Contribute:

Bringing a low-lectin meal not only guarantees that you have something to eat but also lets you share a wonderful and nutritious alternative with others. Bring food that you appreciate and that adheres to your dietary requirements. You'll have at least one assured choice to choose from.

## 3. Focus on the Basics:

Focus on the essentials of a low-lectin diet for social or family gatherings: lean meats, veggies, and healthy fats. Grilled meats, seafood, roasted vegetables, salads, and vegetable-based dishes are all available. Fill your plate with these alternatives to guarantee a nutritious and delicious supper.

## 4. Communicate with Others:

Inform friends, family members, or the host of your dietary requirements if necessary. Explain that you have special food limits for health reasons and respectfully request their understanding and support. Most individuals will be accommodating and want to make you feel at ease.

## 5. Be Prepared with Snacks:

Bring some portable snacks if you anticipate a lack of low-lectin choices. This ensures you have a backup plan in case there are fewer options or items that are incompatible with your diet. Nuts, seeds, fresh fruits, and homemade low-lectin energy snacks can all help you stay satiated.

## 6. Focus on Socializing:

While food is typically an important element of social events, try to focus on the social aspect rather than the meal alone. Participate in activities, engage in conversations, and enjoy the company of loved ones to make the celebration more pleasurable and satisfying.

## 7. Practice Mindful Eating:

Practice mindful eating by paying attention to your body's hunger and fullness cues when choosing meals. Slow down, appreciate the flavors, and pay attention to your body's cues. This will assist you in avoiding overeating and making deliberate decisions that are in line with your dietary requirements.

## 8. Be Flexible:

While sticking to your low-lectin diet is vital, it's also

necessary to be adaptable and understanding in some instances. If you find yourself in a scenario with few options, make the best decisions you can and focus on preserving long-term balance rather than worrying about one specific incident.

## Staying Motivated and Overcoming Setbacks

It is critical for long-term success to stay motivated and overcome difficulties on your low-lectin diet path. Here are some tips to help you stay motivated and recover from setbacks:

**1. Establish Specific Goals:** Set specific and attainable goals for your low-lectin diet. Having defined goals will give direction and motivation, whether it's improving digestion, lowering inflammation, or reaching overall improved health. To stay focused, write down your goals and reread them on a frequent basis.

**2. Educate Yourself:** Continue to study about the advantages of a low-lectin diet and how it may improve your health. To keep your motivation strong, stay up-to-date on the newest research, success stories, and recipes. The more you comprehend the advantages, the more driven you will be to continue.

**3. Recognize and enjoy your tiny successes**: along the way. Celebrate your successes, whether it's effectively avoiding high-lectin meals for a week or attempting a new low-lectin dish. These accomplishments add to your total improvement. Recognizing your efforts will keep you motivated and on track.

**4. Find Support:** Make contact with individuals who are on a low-lectin diet or seeking improved health. Join online networks, support groups, or forums to share your experiences, get advice, and be encouraged. A strong support network may give inspiration, accountability, and a sense of belonging.

**5. Monitor Your Progress:** Keep a notebook or use a tracking tool to keep track of your progress. Document your feelings, health improvements, energy levels, and any good changes you've noticed. Tracking your progress can remind you why you started and inspire you to continue, especially during difficult times.

**6. Incorporate Self-Care into Your Routine:** Take care of your general well-being by adding self-care routines to your routine. Engage in activities that promote relaxation, stress reduction, and mood enhancement. This might include things like exercise, meditation, getting enough sleep, or engaging in hobbies that you enjoy.

**7. Learn from Mistakes:** Mistakes are a normal part of any journey, including a low-lectin diet. Instead of concentrating on defeats, consider them learning experiences. Consider what caused the setback, identify potential triggers, and plan how to avoid such circumstances in the future. Take failures as an opportunity to learn and strengthen your determination.

**8. Maintain a happy Attitude and Be Flexible:** Maintain a happy attitude and be flexible with yourself. Understand that you may depart from your low-lectin diet owing to unforeseen circumstances. Instead of being disheartened, focus on your accomplishments and recommit to your goals. Rather than aiming for perfection, embrace the journey as a process of constant progress.

# CHAPTER NINE

# ADDITIONAL LIFESTYLE CONSIDERATIONS

## Stress Management and Sleep

Stress management and enough sleep are critical for general health, including the effectiveness of your low-lectin diet. Here are some tips to help you manage stress and prioritize good sleep:

**Stress Management:**

**1. Recognize Stress Triggers:** Recognize the events, people, or activities in your life that tend to produce stress. Understanding your stress triggers might help you manage and cope with them better.

**2. Use Relaxation Techniques:** Try relaxation techniques like deep breathing exercises, meditation, yoga, or mindfulness. These techniques can help you relax, lower stress hormones, and create a sense of peace.

**3. Regular Exercises:** Engage in regular physical exercise to release endorphins, which are natural stress-fighting chemicals. Choose activities that you love, such as walking, running, dancing, or yoga, and include them in your daily routine.

**4. Make Self-Care a Priority:** Set aside time each day for self-care activities that offer you joy and relaxation. Reading, having a bath, listening to music, practicing a hobby, or spending quality time with loved ones are all examples.

**5. Establish limits:** To avoid excessive stress, set limits with your job, relationships, and other responsibilities. Learn to say no when required and prioritize activities that are beneficial to your health.

**6. Seek Help:** Seek emotional assistance from friends, family, or a support network. Talking about your anxieties and problems with someone might give you perspective, validation, and viable answers.

**7. Time Management:** Good time management might help you minimize stress. Prioritize your work, delegate as much as is feasible, and divide larger jobs into smaller, more manageable chunks. This might help you feel more in control and less overwhelmed.

**Quality Sleep:**

**1. Establish a constant Sleep routine**: Establish a constant sleep routine by going to bed and getting up at the same time every day, including on weekends. This improves sleep quality by regulating your body's internal clock.

**2. Create a Relaxing Environment:** Make your bedroom sleep-friendly by keeping it cold, dark, and quiet. If required, use blackout curtains, earplugs, or white noise machines. Consider purchasing a suitable mattress and pillows to meet your sleep requirements.

**3. Create a Bedtime Routine:** Relax before bedtime by doing things like reading, having a warm bath, stretching gently, or listening to soothing music. Creating a nighttime ritual alerts your body that it is time to sleep.

**4. Limit Stimulants:** Caffeine, nicotine, and alcohol should be avoided close to bedtime since they can disrupt sleep quality. Instead, choose herbal teas or decaffeinated options.

**5. Disconnect from Screens:** Limit your exposure to electronic devices such as cellphones, tablets, and televisions at least an hour before going to bed. The blue light emitted by screens has the potential to interrupt your sleep-wake cycle. Instead, participate in relaxation-promoting activities.

**6. Manage Bedroom stressors:** Address any bedroom stresses that may interfere with your sleep, such as unpleasant temperatures, sounds, or an uncomfortable mattress. Make changes to create a calm sleeping environment.

**7. Regular Exercise:** Physical activity on a regular basis might enhance sleep quality. Aim for 30 minutes of moderate activity most days of the week, but avoid severe exercise too close to bedtime because it may excite your body.

### Exercise and Physical Activity

Exercise and physical exercise are vital components of a healthy lifestyle and help promote general well-being in addition to a low-lectin diet. Exercise provides various physical and mental health advantages. Consider the following crucial points:

**1. Physical Health Advantages:** Weight Management: Regular exercise aids in weight management by burning calories and raising metabolism. When paired with a healthy diet, it can help you lose weight. Exercise increases cardiovascular fitness, strengthens the heart and blood vessels, and lowers the risk of heart disease, high blood pressure, and stroke.

Weight-bearing workouts like walking, running, and weightlifting help grow and maintain healthy bones, lowering the risk of osteoporosis and fractures. Resistance exercise and weightlifting improve muscular strength and endurance, enhancing overall physical performance and lowering the risk of age-related muscle loss.

- Flexibility and Mobility: Stretching exercises and activities such as yoga and Pilates help increase flexibility, joint range of motion, and general mobility.
- Energy Boost: Regular exercise boosts energy levels, improves stamina, and promotes better sleep, resulting in more energy throughout the day.

## 2. Mental Health Advantages:

- Stress Relief: Exercise increases the synthesis of endorphins, which enhance mood and lower stress levels.
- Better Cognitive Function: Physical activity improves cognitive function, memory, and

attention. It has the potential to lower the risk of cognitive decline and enhance overall brain health.

- Mood Enhancement: Exercise stimulates the release of neurotransmitters such as serotonin and dopamine, which contribute to enhanced mood and a reduction in sadness and anxiety symptoms.

- Improved Sleep: Regular exercise can help regulate sleep patterns, increase sleep quality, and alleviate symptoms of insomnia.

- Boosted Self-Esteem: Achieving fitness objectives and feeling physically stronger may enhance self-esteem and general self-confidence.

**3. Types of Exercise:** Aerobic Exercise: Activities that raise heart rate and breathing, such as brisk walking, jogging, cycling, swimming, or dancing, give

cardiovascular advantages as well as respiratory system strengthening.

- Strength Training: Resistance activities, such as weightlifting or bodyweight workouts, help

  increase muscular strength, boost metabolism, and improve general physical function.

Stretching, yoga, tai chi, and balance training exercises promote flexibility and joint mobility while decreasing the chance of falling.

- Active Lifestyle: Participating in everyday tasks such as gardening, housekeeping, or using the stairs instead of the elevator helps to increase total physical activity levels.

**4. Safety Considerations:** Begin cautiously and progressively to avoid harm. Listen to your body, and don't push yourself too far.

- Select things that you love and alter your routine to keep it interesting and avoid monotony.
- Stay hydrated, wear suitable footwear and clothes, and think about warming up and cooling down before and after workouts.

## Other Complementary Health Practices

Aside from a low-lectin diet and regular exercise, there are a range of alternative health activities that might improve overall health. These practices focus on various aspects of health, including mental, emotional, and physical well-being. Here are two such examples:

**1. Herbal medicines and Supplements:** When used correctly and under the supervision of a healthcare practitioner, herbal medicines and supplements can augment a low-lectin diet. Certain herbs and supplements may provide particular health advantages, such as lowering inflammation, boosting immune function, or enhancing digestion. To guarantee safety and efficacy, it is critical to speak with a healthcare expert.

**2.Breathing techniques:**

Deep breathing techniques, such as diaphragmatic breathing or alternate nostril breathing, can help decrease stress, increase relaxation, and enhance general well-being. These procedures are straightforward, can be performed anywhere, and may be incorporated into regular activities.

**3.Aromatherapy:**

Aromatherapy is the use of essential oils obtained from plants to enhance physical and emotional well-being. Essential oils can be diffused, used topically (dilution is required), or added to baths. Oils contain different characteristics and fragrances that can improve mood, relaxation, and general wellbeing.

**4. Mindfulness and meditation:** Meditation is training the mind to create a state of quiet and focused awareness. It can aid with stress reduction, focus, emotional well-being, and self-awareness. The practice of mindfulness, a type of meditation, involves paying attention to the present moment without judgment. Regular meditation and mindfulness practice can benefit one's overall mental health.

**5. Yoga:** Yoga promotes physical strength, flexibility, and mental well-being by combining physical postures (asanas), breath control (pranayama), and meditation. Yoga practice on a regular basis can help to improve posture, promote body awareness, reduce tension, and improve relaxation.

**6. Acupuncture:** Acupuncture is an ancient Chinese treatment in which fine needles are inserted into precise spots on the body. It is thought to aid in the balance of energy (qi) and facilitate healing. Acupuncture is frequently used to relieve pain, decrease tension, and enhance general well-being.

**7.Massage therapy:** Massage therapy is the manipulation of the soft tissues of the body in order to increase circulation, reduce muscular tension, and induce relaxation. It can aid with stress reduction, pain relief, flexibility, and general physical and mental well-being.

**8. Mind-Body Practices:** Other mind-body practices, such as Tai Chi, Qigong, and Reiki, concentrate on the relationship between the mind, body, and energy flow. These activities seek to create balance, harmony, and energy, and when followed on a daily basis, they can help with general well-being.

# CONCLUSION

In conclusion, the book "The Low Lectin Diet" offers valuable insights and guidance for individuals seeking to improve their health and well-being through dietary choices. Throughout the book, the author explores the concept of lectins, a type of protein found in many plant-based foods, and their potential impact on our bodies.

The book begins by explaining lectins, their role in plants, and their possible implications on human health. It delves into the numerous lectin sources in our diets, highlighting typical foods that are high in these proteins. By digging into the science of lectins, the author empowers readers with the knowledge they need to make educated dietary decisions.

"The Low Lectin Diet" then provides a step-by-step guide to adopting a low-lectin diet. It provides a detailed list of items to include and avoid, emphasizing the significance of a varied and balanced diet. The book also includes practical suggestions and tactics for navigating grocery shopping, meal planning, and dining out while keeping to the low-lectin guidelines.

One of the book's most noticeable qualities is its emphasis on evidence-based material. Throughout the chapters, the author cites scientific studies and research to back up his statements concerning lectins and their possible consequences. By offering this scientific foundation, the book provides readers with a sense of trustworthiness and confidence, helping them to make well-informed judgments regarding their food choices.

Furthermore, "The Low Lectin Diet" goes beyond a mere collection of guidelines and recipes. It dives into the potential benefits of adopting a low-lectin diet, such as improved digestion, reduced inflammation, and enhanced overall health. The author acknowledges that individual responses may vary and encourages readers to listen to their bodies and make adjustments accordingly.

It is important to highlight, however, that the book reflects just one point of view on nutrition and health. While the low-lectin diet may be useful for some people, it may not be appropriate or essential for everyone. Before making substantial dietary changes, it is usually best to talk with a healthcare practitioner or certified dietician.

In conclusion, "The Low Lectin Diet" provides a thorough and instructive guide to understanding lectins and adopting dietary choices that match with a low-lectin lifestyle. The book enables readers to take charge of their health and make educated dietary decisions by providing evidence-based knowledge, practical techniques, and potential rewards. Whether or whether one decides to follow a low-lectin diet, this book is a useful resource for anybody interested in learning more about the influence of nutrition on well-being.